Carb Cycling for Beginners

Easy-to-follow Recipes and Exercises to Lose Weight, Build Muscles, and Stay Healthy

Chandler La Rocca

Table of Contents

Introduction

Carb Cycling for Beginners

Welcome to "Carb Cycling for Beginners: Easy-to-follow Recipes and Exercises to Lose Weight, Build Muscles, and Stay Healthy." In this introduction, we'll provide an overview of the key elements that you can expect to find in this book and why they are important for your journey to better health and fitness.

Explanation of Carb Cycling and Its Benefits

Carb cycling is a nutritional strategy that has gained popularity among fitness enthusiasts and those seeking to manage their weight effectively. It involves alternating between days of varying carbohydrate intake to optimize your body's performance and to achieve specific fitness goals. The key benefits of carb cycling include:

- **Weight Management:** Carb cycling can help you lose excess body fat while preserving muscle mass, making it an effective tool for both weight loss and muscle definition.
- **Improved Energy Levels:** By strategically adjusting your carb intake, you can optimize your energy levels for workouts and daily activities.
- **Enhanced Metabolism:** Carb cycling can help prevent metabolic adaptation, which often occurs with long-term calorie restriction, by varying your intake of macronutrients.
- **Sustainable and Flexible:** This approach is adaptable to your lifestyle and preferences, making it easier to maintain over the long term.

How the Book is Structured

This book is designed to be your comprehensive guide to carb cycling, providing you with practical information, easy-to-follow recipes, and effective exercises. It is divided into three parts, each focusing on different levels of carbohydrate intake: Low Carb, Moderate Carb, and High Carb. Within each part, you will find dedicated sections for Breakfast, Lunch, Dinner, Snacks, and Desserts.

The structure of each section is consistent, with detailed ingredient lists, step-by-step instructions, total calorie counts, and estimated preparation times for each recipe. This ensures that you have everything you need to create delicious and nutritious meals that align with your carb cycling goals.

The book also includes a 30-day meal plan to help you get started, complete with exercises and workout plans tailored to each phase of carb cycling.

The Importance of a Balanced Approach to Nutrition and Exercise

While carb cycling is a powerful tool, it is essential to remember that it is just one part of the equation. To achieve your health and fitness goals, it is crucial to maintain a balanced approach that encompasses not only your dietary choices but also your physical activity.

In this book, we emphasize the importance of combining your carb cycling plan with a well-rounded fitness routine. This holistic approach ensures that you are not only optimizing your nutrition but also promoting overall wellness. We provide guidance on exercise routines that complement your carb cycling phases, ensuring that your efforts yield the best results.

Setting Realistic Goals

One of the keys to success in any fitness and nutrition journey is setting achievable and realistic goals. We encourage you to define clear and attainable objectives that will guide your carb cycling plan. Whether you're looking to shed extra pounds, build lean muscle, or enhance your overall well-being, having clear goals will keep you motivated and on track.

Throughout the book, we offer guidance on goal setting and how to tailor your carb cycling plan to align with your unique aspirations.

By incorporating these key principles of carb cycling, structured meal plans, and comprehensive exercise guidance, "Carb Cycling for Beginners" equips you with the knowledge and tools necessary to embark on achieving your exercise and health objectives with success. So, let's get started on your path to a healthier, stronger, and happier you.

Part 1: Low Carb Recipes and Exercises

Welcome to the first part of "Carb Cycling for Beginners." In this section, we will focus on low carb days, providing you with a variety of delicious recipes and effective exercises to help you make the most of this phase of your carb cycling journey.

Chapter 1

Low Carb Basics

Welcome to the first chapter of "Carb Cycling for Beginners." In this chapter, we will explore the fundamental concepts of low carb days, setting the stage for your carb cycling journey.

Explanation of Low Carb Days

Low carb days are a crucial component of carb cycling, a dietary strategy that alternates between periods of high and low carbohydrate consumption. On low carb days, your goal is to restrict your daily carbohydrate intake significantly compared to your regular diet. The primary purpose of incorporating low carb days is to encourage your body to shift from using carbohydrates as its primary energy source to relying on stored fat. This shift promotes fat loss and helps maintain muscle mass.

During low carb days, you aim to consume fewer carbohydrates to deplete glycogen stores in your muscles and liver. This state of glycogen depletion triggers the body to tap into fat stores for energy. Low carb days are usually interspersed with moderate and high carb days to strike a balance between fat loss and muscle preservation, creating an effective approach for achieving your fitness and weight management goals.

Recommended Food Sources

For successful execution of low carb days, it is essential to choose the right foods. The following is a list of recommended food sources for low carb days:

- **Lean Proteins:** Include sources such as chicken, turkey, lean beef, fish, and tofu. These provide essential amino acids and help preserve muscle mass during low carb days.
- **Healthy Fats:** Incorporate sources like avocados, nuts, seeds, olive oil, and fatty fish. These fats are satiating and provide a source of energy.
- **Non-Starchy Vegetables:** Choose vegetables such as leafy greens, broccoli, cauliflower, and bell peppers. These are low in carbohydrates and rich in fiber and vitamins.

- **Low-Carb Fruits:** Opt for fruits like berries, which are lower in carbohydrates compared to tropical fruits like bananas and mangoes.
- **Dairy Products:** Include plain Greek yogurt and cheese in moderation, as they provide protein and healthy fats with relatively fewer carbs.
- **Eggs:** Eggs are an excellent source of protein and healthy fats, making them a versatile option for low carb meals.

By incorporating these foods into your low carb meals, you can maintain satiety, support muscle preservation, and effectively manage your weight.

Benefits of Low Carb Cycling

Embracing low carb days offers several benefits to individuals who are looking to optimize their nutrition and achieve their fitness goals:

- **Weight Loss:** Low carb days create a calorie deficit, making them an effective strategy for shedding excess body fat.
- **Blood Sugar Control:** Reducing carbohydrate intake can help stabilize blood sugar levels and improve insulin sensitivity.
- **Reduced Inflammation:** Some individuals experience decreased inflammation and water retention on low carb days.
- **Enhanced Fat Burn:** Glycogen depletion encourages the body to rely on fat stores for energy, facilitating fat loss.

How to Calculate Your Daily Carb Intake

Personalizing your low carb intake is essential to maximize the benefits of low carb days. We will guide you through the process of calculating your daily carbohydrate intake based on your specific goals, activity level, and body composition. This tailored approach ensures that you can harness the full potential of low carb days and optimize your progress.

With a solid understanding of the basics of low carb days, you are well-equipped to explore the low carb recipes and exercises that follow in subsequent chapters. These foundational principles lay the groundwork for your carb cycling journey, allowing you to harness the full potential of this approach to reach your fitness and health objectives.

Chapter 2

Low Carb Breakfast Recipes

In this chapter, we've curated a selection of low carb breakfast recipes that are not only delicious but also easy to prepare. Each recipe is designed to keep you feeling satisfied and energized, making it a perfect start to your low carb day.

Spinach and Feta Omelette

Ingredients:

- 2 large eggs
- 1 cup fresh spinach, chopped
- 2 tablespoons crumbled feta cheese
- Salt and pepper to taste
- Cooking spray

Instructions:

1. Heat a non-stick skillet over medium-high heat and coat with cooking spray.
2. Whisk the eggs in a bowl and season with salt and pepper.
3. Pour the whisked eggs into the skillet, swirling to ensure even coverage.
4. Add the chopped spinach and crumbled feta cheese evenly across the eggs.
5. Cook for 2-3 minutes until the edges set, then fold the omelette in half.
6. Cook for an additional 1-2 minutes until the center is no longer runny.
7. Transfer the omelette to a serving platter and serve.

Total Calories:

- Approximately 280 calories

Preparation Time:

- 10 minutes

Chia Seed Pudding with Berries

Ingredients:

- 2 tablespoons chia seeds
- 1/2 cup unsweetened almond milk
- 1/2 teaspoon vanilla extract
- 1/2 cup of mixed berries, including raspberries, blueberries, and strawberries
- 1 teaspoon honey (optional)

Instructions:

1. In a jar or bowl, combine chia seeds, almond milk, and vanilla extract.
2. Stir well to disperse the chia seeds evenly.
3. Cover the container and refrigerate for at least 2 hours or overnight, allowing the chia seeds to absorb the liquid and create a pudding-like texture.
4. Before serving, top the chia pudding with mixed berries and a drizzle of honey if desired.

Total Calories:

- Approximately 200 calories

Preparation Time:

- 5 minutes (plus chilling time)

Chia Seed Pudding with Berries

Avocado and Bacon Breakfast Salad

Ingredients:

- 1 ripe avocado, diced
- 2 cooked and crumbled bacon slices
- 2 hard-boiled eggs, sliced
- 1 cup of mixed greens (arugula, spinach, etc.)
- Salt and pepper to taste
- 1 tablespoon olive oil
- 1 teaspoon balsamic vinegar

Instructions:

1. In a bowl, combine the diced avocado, crumbled bacon, sliced hard-boiled eggs, and mixed greens.
2. Drizzle with olive oil and balsamic vinegar.
3. To taste, add salt and pepper for seasoning.
4. Toss gently to combine, and serve.

Total Calories:

- Approximately 350 calories

Preparation Time:

- 15 minutes

These low carb breakfast recipes are not only easy to make but also packed with flavor and nutrients, ensuring that you start your day with energy and satisfaction while staying on track with your carb cycling plan. Enjoy a variety of these breakfast options throughout your low carb days.

Chapter 3

Low Carb Lunch Recipes

Lunch is a significant meal in your low carb day, and it's important to choose satisfying and delicious options. In this chapter, you'll find a collection of low carb lunch recipes to keep you on track with your carb cycling plan.

Grilled Chicken Caesar Salad

Ingredients:

- 4 oz grilled chicken breast, sliced
- 2 cups romaine lettuce, chopped
- 2 tablespoons Caesar salad dressing (low-carb)
- 1 tablespoon grated Parmesan cheese
- Croutons (optional, use low-carb alternatives)
- Salt and pepper to taste

Instructions:

1. In a large bowl, combine the chopped romaine lettuce, grilled chicken slices, and croutons (if using).
2. Drizzle the Caesar salad dressing over the salad and toss to coat.
3. To taste, add salt and pepper for seasoning.
4. Sprinkle the grated Parmesan cheese on top before serving.

Total Calories:

- Approximately 350 calories

Preparation Time:

- 15 minutes

Turkey and Avocado Lettuce Wraps

Ingredients:

- 4 large lettuce leaves (e.g., iceberg or Romaine)
- 4 oz lean turkey slices
- 1 avocado, sliced
- 1/4 red onion, thinly sliced
- 2 tablespoons Greek yogurt or sour cream (low-carb)
- 1 teaspoon hot sauce (optional)
- Salt and pepper to taste

Instructions:

1. Arrange the lettuce leaves on a clean surface.
2. Layer each lettuce leaf with turkey slices, avocado slices, and red onion.
3. In a small bowl, mix Greek yogurt (or sour cream) and hot sauce (if using).
4. Drizzle the yogurt sauce over the lettuce wraps.
5. To taste, add salt and pepper for seasoning.
6. Carefully fold the lettuce leaves over the filling to create wraps.
7. Serve and enjoy.

Total Calories:

- Approximately 320 calories

Preparation Time:

- 10 minutes

Zucchini Noodles with Pesto

Ingredients:

- 2 medium zucchinis, spiralized into noodles
- 2 tablespoons pesto sauce (low-carb)
- 1/4 cup cherry tomatoes, halved
- 2 tablespoons grated Parmesan cheese
- Fresh basil leaves for garnish
- Salt and pepper to taste

Instructions:

1. In a skillet, heat a bit of olive oil over medium heat.
2. Add the zucchini noodles and sauté for 2-3 minutes until tender but not overcooked.
3. Remove the skillet from heat and add the pesto sauce, tossing to coat the noodles.
4. To taste, add salt and pepper for seasoning.
5. Transfer the zucchini noodles to a serving plate.
6. Top with halved cherry tomatoes, grated Parmesan cheese, and fresh basil leaves.
7. Serve warm.

Total Calories:

- Approximately 280 calories

Preparation Time:

- 15 minutes

These low carb lunch recipes are not only low in carbohydrates but also rich in flavor and nutrients. Enjoy these options to keep your energy levels up and your carb intake on track during your low carb days.

Chapter 4

Low Carb Dinner Recipes

Dinner is another crucial meal during your low carb days. These low carb dinner recipes are designed to help you finish your day strong while sticking to your carb cycling plan.

Baked Salmon with Asparagus

Ingredients:

- 6 oz salmon fillet
- 1/2 bunch of asparagus, trimmed
- 1 tablespoon olive oil
- 1 lemon, sliced
- 1 teaspoon garlic powder
- Salt and pepper to taste

Instructions:

1. Preheat your oven to 375°F (190°C).
2. Place the asparagus on a baking sheet and drizzle with olive oil.
3. Sprinkle with garlic powder, salt, and pepper, then toss to coat.
4. Lay the salmon fillet on the baking sheet, skin-side down.
5. Season the salmon with salt, pepper, and a few lemon slices.
6. Bake for 15-20 minutes, or until the salmon flakes easily with a fork and the asparagus is tender.
7. Serve with additional lemon slices for extra flavor.

Total Calories:

- Approximately 380 calories

Preparation Time:

- 25 minutes

Spaghetti Squash with Marinara Sauce

Ingredients:

- 1 medium spaghetti squash
- 1 cup low-carb marinara sauce
- 1/4 cup grated Parmesan cheese
- Fresh basil leaves for garnish
- Salt and pepper to taste

Instructions:

1. Preheat your oven to 375°F (190°C).
2. Scoop out the seeds of the spaghetti squash by cutting it in half lengthwise.
3. Place the squash halves on a baking pan, cut side down.
4. Bake for 30-40 minutes, or until the flesh is tender and easily scraped into "noodles" with a fork.
5. Heat the marinara sauce in a saucepan.
6. Scrape the spaghetti squash flesh into a serving dish.
7. Pour the marinara sauce over the "noodles."
8. Sprinkle with grated Parmesan cheese and fresh basil leaves.
9. Season with salt and pepper to taste.

Total Calories:

Approximately 250 calories

Preparation Time:

50 minutes

Beef and Broccoli Stir-Fry

Ingredients:

- 6 oz beef sirloin, thinly sliced
- 2 cups broccoli florets
- 1 clove garlic, minced
- 2 tablespoons low-sodium soy sauce
- 1 tablespoon olive oil
- 1/2 teaspoon ginger, minced
- Sesame seeds for garnish (optional)
- Salt and pepper to taste

Instructions:

1. In a wok or large skillet, heat the olive oil over medium-high heat.
2. Add the minced garlic and ginger and sauté for 1 minute.
3. Add the beef slices and stir-fry for 3-4 minutes or until they're cooked to your desired level of doneness. Take out and put aside the steak from the pan.
4. In the same pan, add the broccoli florets and stir-fry for about 5 minutes until they're tender-crisp.
5. Return the cooked beef to the pan and add the soy sauce.
6. Toss to combine and cook for an additional 2 minutes.
7. To taste, add salt and pepper for seasoning.
8. Sprinkle with sesame seeds for extra flavor and garnish.

Total Calories:

- Approximately 320 calories

Preparation Time:

- 20 minutes

These low carb dinner recipes offer a satisfying end to your low carb day while ensuring you stay on track with your carb cycling plan. Enjoy the flavors, and stay committed to your health and fitness goals.

Chapter 5

Low Carb Snack Recipes

Snacking can be a challenge on low carb days, but these low carb snack recipes are designed to keep your energy levels stable and curb your cravings while staying within your carb cycling plan.

Cucumber and Hummus

Ingredients:

- 1 medium cucumber, sliced
- 2 tablespoons of hummus (low-carb)
- Salt and pepper to taste

Instructions:

1. Wash and slice the cucumber into rounds or sticks.
2. Serve with a side of low-carb hummus for dipping.
3. To taste, add salt and pepper for seasoning.

Total Calories:

- Approximately 50 calories

Preparation Time:

- 5 minutes

Almond and Coconut Energy Bites

Ingredients:

- 1/2 cup almond butter (no added sugar)
- 1/4 cup unsweetened shredded coconut
- 2 tablespoons chia seeds
- 1 tablespoon low-carb sweetener (e.g., erythritol, stevia)
- 1/2 teaspoon vanilla extract

Instructions:

1. In a mixing bowl, combine almond butter, shredded coconut, chia seeds, sweetener, and vanilla extract.
2. Stir until the mixture is well combined and sticks together.
3. Form the mixture into bite-sized balls and place them on a baking sheet lined with parchment paper.
4. Refrigerate for at least 30 minutes to firm up the energy bites.
5. Once set, store them in an airtight container for easy snacking.

Total Calories:

Approximately 90 calories per energy bite

Preparation Time:

10 minutes (plus chilling time)

Deviled Eggs

Ingredients:

- 4 hard-boiled eggs
- 2 tablespoons mayonnaise (low-carb)
- 1 teaspoon Dijon mustard
- Paprika for garnish (optional)
- Salt and pepper to taste

Instructions:

1. Split the hard-boiled eggs in half along their length.
2. Carefully remove the yolks and place them in a bowl.
3. Add mayonnaise, Dijon mustard, salt, and pepper to the yolks.
4. Mash and mix until you have a creamy filling.
5. Spoon the filling back into the egg white halves.
6. Sprinkle with paprika for added flavor and garnish.

Total Calories:

- Approximately 80 calories for two halves

Preparation Time:

- 15 minutes

These low carb snack recipes offer variety and flavor to keep you satisfied and fueled between meals on your low carb days. Enjoy these guilt-free options while maintaining your commitment to your carb cycling plan.

Chapter 6

Low Carb Dessert Recipes

Satisfying your sweet tooth on low carb days is possible with these delicious and guilt-free low carb dessert recipes. Enjoy these treats without derailing your carb cycling plan.

Chocolate Avocado Mousse

Ingredients:

- 1 ripe avocado
- 2 tablespoons unsweetened cocoa powder
- 2 tablespoons low-carb sweetener (e.g., stevia, erythritol)
- 1/2 teaspoon vanilla extract
- A pinch of salt
- Whipped cream for garnish (optional)

Instructions:

1. Cut the avocado in half, remove the pit, and scoop out the flesh.
2. In a blender or food processor, combine the avocado, cocoa powder, sweetener, vanilla extract, and a pinch of salt.
3. Blend the ingredients until it becomes creamy and smooth.
4. Taste and add more sweetener if necessary to suit the sweetness.
5. Divide the mousse into serving dishes.
6. If desired, top with a dollop of whipped cream.
7. Place in the refrigerator for at least 30 minutes before serving.

Total Calories:

- Approximately 250 calories

Preparation Time:

- 10 minutes

Berries with Whipped Cream

Ingredients:

- 1/2 cup of berries (strawberries, blueberries, raspberries, etc.)
- 2 tablespoons unsweetened whipped cream
- 1/2 teaspoon low-carb sweetener (optional)

Instructions:

1. Wash and dry the mixed berries.
2. In a serving dish, arrange the berries.
3. If desired, sprinkle with a small amount of low-carb sweetener for added sweetness.
4. Top with a generous dollop of unsweetened whipped cream.
5. Serve and enjoy!

Total Calories:

Approximately 100 calories

Preparation Time:

5 minutes

Berries with Whipped Cream

Keto-Friendly Cheesecake

Ingredients:

- 4 oz cream cheese
- 1/4 cup almond flour
- 2 tablespoons low-carb sweetener (e.g., erythritol)
- 1/2 teaspoon vanilla extract
- A pinch of salt
- 1 egg
- 1 tablespoon melted butter

Instructions:

1. Preheat the oven to 325°F (160°C) and prepare a muffin pan with paper liners.
2. In a mixing bowl, combine cream cheese, almond flour, sweetener, vanilla extract, and a pinch of salt. Mix until smooth.
3. Mix in the egg until fully mixed.
4. Divide the mixture into the muffin tin, filling each cup about two-thirds full.
5. Drizzle melted butter over each cheesecake.
6. Bake for 20-25 minutes or until the edges are set and the centers are slightly jiggly.
7. Allow the mini cheesecakes to cool and set in the fridge for a few hours or overnight.
8. Serve and enjoy your low carb cheesecake.

Total Calories:

Approximately 200 calories per mini cheesecake

Preparation Time:

35 minutes (plus chilling time)

These low carb dessert recipes offer a sweet ending to your low carb day without compromising your carb cycling plan. Enjoy these delectable treats and stay on track with your health and fitness goals.

Chapter 7

Low Carb Exercises

In this chapter, we'll focus on the recommended exercises for your low carb days, providing detailed workout plans and valuable tips to ensure you make the most of your workouts while following your carb cycling plan.

Recommended Exercises for Low Carb Days

Bodyweight Squats:

- Place your feet shoulder-width apart.
- Lower your body by bending your knees and maintaining your back upright.
- Return to your starting position by pressing through your heels.
- Aim for three sets of 15-20 reps.

Plank Variations:

- Standard Plank: Hold a push-up position with your arms straight and your body in a straight line.
- Side Plank: Support your body weight on one forearm, keeping your body straight.
- Plank with Leg Lift: Raise one leg a few inches off the ground while doing a conventional plank.
- Perform each plank variation for 30-60 seconds and repeat 2-3 sets.

Resistance Band Workouts:

- Resistance bands can provide a full-body workout, including exercises like bicep curls, lateral raises, and leg lifts.
- Incorporate resistance band exercises for 15-20 minutes in your low carb day workout routine.

Detailed Workout Plans

Workout 1 - Full Body Bodyweight Circuit:

- Bodyweight Squats: 3 sets of 15-20 reps
- Push-Ups: 3 sets of 10-15 reps
- Plank (Standard): 3 sets of 30-60 seconds
- Rest: 30-45 seconds between sets

Workout 2 - Core and Balance:

- Side Planks (each side): 3 sets of 30-60 seconds
- Plank with Leg Lifts: 3 sets of 30-60 seconds
- Single-Leg Glute Bridge: 3 sets of 10-15 reps per leg
- Rest: 30-45 seconds between sets

Workout 3 - Resistance Band Full-Body Routine:

- Bicep Curls: 3 sets of 12-15 reps
- Lateral Raises: 3 sets of 12-15 reps
- Leg Lifts: three sets of 12-15 reps.
- Rest: 30-45 seconds between sets

Tips for Effective Low Carb Workouts

- **Stay Hydrated:** Dehydration can affect your energy levels and performance. Before, during, and after your exercise, drink lots of water.
- **Prioritize Protein:** Consume a protein-rich snack or meal before your workout to support muscle recovery and minimize muscle breakdown.
- **Warm Up and Cool Down:** Always start with a warm-up to prepare your muscles and finish with a cool-down to prevent stiffness and reduce the risk of injury.
- **Listen to Your Body:** If you're feeling fatigued during a low carb workout, it's okay to reduce the intensity or duration to prevent overexertion.
- **Recovery:** After your workout, consume a post-workout meal that includes protein and carbohydrates to replenish glycogen stores and support muscle recovery.
- **Consistency:** Consistency is key to seeing progress. Stick to your workout routine and adjust it as needed to align with your fitness goals and carb cycling plan.

By incorporating these exercises and following the workout plans, you'll maximize the benefits of your low carb days, maintain your energy levels, and support your overall fitness and health objectives. Staying consistent and making smart choices in your low carb workouts will help you reach your goals more effectively.

Part 2: Moderate Carb Recipes and Exercises

Welcome to the second part of "Carb Cycling for Beginners." In this section, we will explore moderate carb days, providing you with a variety of delicious recipes and effective exercises tailored to this phase of your carb cycling journey.

Chapter 8

Moderate Carb Basics

In this chapter, we'll explore the essential concepts of moderate carb days, providing you with a clear understanding of how this phase fits into your carb cycling journey.

Explanation of Moderate Carb Days

Moderate carb days represent a balanced approach within the carb cycling framework. These days involve consuming a moderate amount of carbohydrates, falling between the low carb and high carb extremes. The goal of moderate carb days is to strike a balance between fat loss and muscle preservation while providing sufficient energy for workouts and daily activities.

On moderate carb days, your carbohydrate intake will be higher than on low carb days but lower than on high carb days. This balance allows your body to replenish glycogen stores, which are essential for energy during physical activities, without promoting excess fat storage.

Recommended Food Sources

To make the most of your moderate carb days, it's crucial to choose the right sources of carbohydrates. Focus on complex carbohydrates from whole, unprocessed foods. Some recommended food sources include:

- **Whole grains:** Brown rice, quinoa, whole wheat pasta, and oats.
- **Starchy vegetables:** Sweet potatoes, butternut squash, and peas.
- **Legumes:** Beans, lentils, and chickpeas.
- **Fruits:** Berries, apples, and citrus fruits.
- **Dairy:** Greek yogurt and milk.
- **Lean proteins:** turkey, fish, tofu, and chicken.

These foods provide a balanced source of nutrients, including carbohydrates, fiber, protein, and healthy fats, ensuring you stay satiated and energized during your moderate carb days.

Benefits of Moderate Carb Cycling

Moderate carb cycling offers a range of benefits:

- **Balanced Energy:** Moderate carb days provide a balance between energy from carbohydrates and fat. This helps you maintain energy levels without causing spikes in insulin.
- **Muscle Preservation:** By consuming a moderate amount of carbohydrates, you support muscle preservation while still promoting fat loss.
- **Sustainability:** Moderate carb days are sustainable in the long term and can be more enjoyable than strict low carb days.
- **Versatility:** The flexibility of moderate carb cycling allows you to adapt your carb intake to your activity level and goals.

How to Calculate Your Daily Carb Intake on Moderate Carb Days

Calculating your daily carbohydrate intake on moderate carb days is essential for tailoring your carb cycling plan to your individual needs. Here's a simplified method:

- Determine your total daily calorie intake for weight maintenance or your specific goal (e.g., weight loss, muscle gain).
- On moderate carb days, aim to allocate about 30-40% of your total calories from carbohydrates. The exact percentage may vary based on your preferences and goals.
- Convert the calories from carbohydrates into grams. Carbohydrates provide approximately 4 calories per gram. For example, if you're consuming 1,800 calories per day, and you want 35% of those calories to come from carbohydrates, it would be $(0.35 * 1,800) / 4 = 157.5$ grams of carbohydrates.

By following these principles, you can personalize your carb intake on moderate carb days to align with your objectives and activity level while maintaining a balanced approach to nutrition and exercise.

Chapter 9

Moderate Carb Breakfast Recipes

A balanced and nutritious breakfast is essential for providing energy and setting the tone for your moderate carb day. Here are some delicious moderate carb breakfast recipes to get you started.

Berry and Yogurt Parfait

Ingredients:

- 1/2 cup Greek yogurt
- 1/2 cup of berries (strawberries, blueberries, raspberries e.t.c)
- 1/4 cup granola (choose a low-sugar, moderate-carb option)
- 1 tablespoon honey (optional)
- A sprinkle of chia seeds

Instructions:

1. Arrange granola, mixed berries, and Greek yogurt in a glass or dish.
2. Drizzle with honey for extra sweetness if desired.
3. Top with a sprinkle of chia seeds for added texture and nutrients.

Total Calories:

- Approximately 350 calories

Preparation Time:

- 5 minutes

Veggie Omelette

Ingredients:

- 2 large eggs
- 1/4 cup bell peppers, diced
- 1/4 cup spinach, chopped
- 1/4 cup diced tomatoes
- 1/4 cup shredded cheese (choose a moderate-carb cheese)
- Salt and pepper to taste

Instructions:

1. In a bowl, whisk the eggs and season with salt and pepper.
2. Spray a nonstick skillet with cooking spray and heat over medium heat.
3. Add the diced peppers, spinach, and tomatoes to the skillet and sauté for a few minutes until softened.
4. Pour the whisked eggs over the veggies in the skillet.
5. Sprinkle the shredded cheese on top.
6. Cook until the edges are set and the center is no longer runny.
7. Fold the omelette in half and slide it onto a plate.

Total Calories:

- Approximately 400 calories

Preparation Time:

- 10 minutes

Whole Grain Pancakes

Ingredients:

- 1/2 cup whole wheat flour
- 1/2 teaspoon baking powder
- 1 tbsp low-carb sweetener (such as stevia or erythritol)
- 1/2 cup almond milk
- 1 egg
- 1/2 teaspoon vanilla extract

Instructions:

1. In a bowl, mix whole wheat flour, baking powder, and sweetener.
2. In another bowl, whisk together almond milk, egg, and vanilla extract.
3. Combine the wet and dry ingredients and stir until you have a smooth batter.
4. Apply cooking spray to a nonstick skillet and place it over medium heat.
5. Pour 1/4 cup batter into the griddle for each pancake.
6. Cook until bubbles appear on the top, then turn and cook until golden brown.
7. Serve with a moderate amount of low-sugar syrup or fresh berries.

Total Calories:

Approximately 350 calories

Preparation Time:

15 minutes

These moderate carb breakfast recipes offer a balance of carbohydrates, protein, and healthy fats to keep you satisfied and energized throughout the morning while maintaining your carb cycling plan. Enjoy a variety of these breakfast options during your moderate carb days.

Chapter 10

Moderate Carb Lunch Recipes

Lunch provides an opportunity to enjoy flavorful meals with the right balance of carbohydrates to support your moderate carb days. Here are some delicious moderate carb lunch recipes for you to try.

Quinoa and Black Bean Salad

Ingredients:

- 1 cup cooked quinoa
- 1/2 cup black beans, drained and rinsed
- 1/4 cup corn kernels
- 1/4 cup diced bell peppers (red, green, or yellow)
- 1/4 cup cherry tomatoes, halved
- 2 tablespoons fresh cilantro, chopped
- Juice of 1 lime
- 1 tablespoon olive oil
- Salt and pepper to taste

Instructions:

1. In a large bowl, combine cooked quinoa, black beans, corn, diced bell peppers, cherry tomatoes, and chopped cilantro.
2. In a separate small bowl, whisk together the lime juice, olive oil, salt, and pepper to create the dressing.
3. Pour the salad with the dressing and toss to mix.
4. Serve chilled.

Total Calories:

Approximately 400 calories

Preparation Time:

20 minutes

Grilled Chicken and Vegetable Wrap

Ingredients:

- 4 oz grilled chicken breast, sliced
- 1 whole-grain tortilla or wrap
- 1/4 cup hummus (choose a moderate-carb variety)
- 1/2 cup mixed greens (e.g., spinach, arugula)
- 1/4 cup sliced cucumbers
- 1/4 cup diced red onions
- 1/4 cup diced tomatoes
- Salt and pepper to taste

Instructions:

1. Lay out the whole-grain tortilla or wrap.
2. Spread hummus on top of the tortilla.
3. Place the sliced grilled chicken on top of the hummus.
4. Add mixed greens, cucumbers, red onions, and diced tomatoes.
5. To taste, add salt and pepper for seasoning.
6. Fold the tortilla in half, then present it.

Total Calories:

- Approximately 450 calories

Preparation Time:

- 15 minutes

Salmon and Asparagus Quiche

Ingredients:

- 4 oz cooked salmon, flaked
- 1 cup asparagus spears, blanched and chopped
- 4 large eggs
- 1/2 cup low-fat milk
- 1/2 cup shredded cheese (choose a moderate-carb variety)
- 1/4 cup chopped fresh dill
- Salt and pepper to taste

Instructions:

1. Preheat your oven to 350°F (175°C) and grease a quiche or pie dish.
2. In a mixing bowl, combine the flaked salmon and chopped asparagus.
3. In another bowl, whisk together the eggs, milk, shredded cheese, and chopped dill. Season with salt and pepper.
4. Pour the egg mixture over the salmon and asparagus in the quiche dish.
5. Bake for 25-30 minutes or until the quiche is set and lightly browned.
6. Let it cool somewhat before slicing and serving.

Total Calories:

- Approximately 380 calories

Preparation Time:

- 40 minutes

These moderate carb lunch recipes offer a balance of carbohydrates, protein, and fiber to keep you satisfied and energized throughout the day while maintaining your carb cycling plan. Enjoy a variety of these lunch options during your moderate carb days.

Chapter 11

Moderate Carb Dinner Recipes

Dinner is an opportunity to enjoy a satisfying and balanced meal on your moderate carb days. Here are some delicious moderate carb dinner recipes for you to explore.

Lemon Herb Grilled Chicken

Ingredients:

- 6 oz chicken breast
- 1 lemon, juiced and zested
- 2 cloves garlic, minced
- 1 tablespoon fresh rosemary, chopped
- 1 tablespoon fresh thyme, chopped
- Salt and pepper to taste
- 1 cup quinoa, cooked (for serving)
- Steamed broccoli (as a side)

Instructions:

1. In a bowl, combine lemon juice, lemon zest, minced garlic, chopped rosemary, and thyme.
2. Season the chicken breast with salt and pepper, then brush the lemon herb mixture over the chicken.
3. Turn the heat up to medium-high on a grill or grill pan.
4. Grill the chicken for about 6-8 minutes per side, or until it's no longer pink in the center.
5. Serve the grilled chicken over a bed of cooked quinoa and with a side of steamed broccoli.

Total Calories:

- Approximately 450 calories

Preparation Time:

- 30 minutes

Shrimp and Broccoli Stir-Fry

Ingredients:

- 6 oz shrimp, peeled and deveined
- 2 cups broccoli florets
- 1 bell pepper, sliced
- 2 cloves garlic, minced
- 1/4 cup low-sodium soy sauce
- 1 tablespoon honey (or low-carb sweetener)
- 1 tablespoon sesame oil
- 1 teaspoon ginger, minced
- Cooked brown rice (for serving)

Instructions:

1. In a small bowl, whisk together the soy sauce, honey, sesame oil, and minced ginger to create the stir-fry sauce.
2. In a large skillet, heat a bit of olive oil over medium-high heat.
3. Add the shrimp and cook for 2-3 minutes on each side until they turn pink and opaque. After taking the shrimp out of the pan, put them aside.
4. In the same skillet, add the garlic, bell pepper, and broccoli. Stir-fry for 5 minutes, or until the veggies are tender-crisp.
5. Return the cooked shrimp to the skillet and pour the stir-fry sauce over the ingredients.
6. Toss to combine and cook for an additional 2 minutes.
7. Serve the shrimp and vegetable stir-fry over cooked brown rice.

Total Calories:

- Approximately 400 calories

Preparation Time:

- 20 minutes

Vegetarian Stuffed Bell Peppers

Ingredients:

- 2 large bell peppers, halved and seeds removed
- 1 cup cooked quinoa
- 1/2 cup black beans, drained and rinsed
- 1/2 cup corn kernels
- 1/2 cup diced tomatoes
- 1/4 cup shredded cheese (choose a moderate-carb variety)
- 1/2 teaspoon chili powder
- Salt and pepper to taste

Instructions:

1. Preheat your oven to 375°F (190°C).
2. In a bowl, combine cooked quinoa, black beans, corn, diced tomatoes, shredded cheese, chili powder, salt, and pepper.
3. Fill the halved bell peppers with the quinoa mixture.
4. Place the stuffed bell peppers in a baking dish.
5. Cover the dish with foil and bake for 25-30 minutes or until the bell peppers are tender.
6. Remove the foil and bake for an additional 5 minutes until the cheese is bubbly and slightly golden.

Total Calories:

- Approximately 380 calories

Preparation Time:

- 45 minutes

These moderate carb dinner recipes offer a balance of carbohydrates, protein, and nutrients to keep you satisfied and energized during your moderate carb days. Enjoy these dinner options as you maintain your commitment to your carb cycling plan.

Chapter 12

Moderate Carb Snack Recipes

Enjoying nutritious and balanced snacks on your moderate carb days can help maintain your energy levels and keep you on track with your carb cycling plan. Here are some delicious moderate carb snack recipes to satisfy your cravings.

Greek Yogurt and Fruit Parfait

Ingredients:

- 1/2 cup Greek yogurt
- 1/2 cup of berries (strawberries, blueberries, raspberries e.t.c)
- 1/4 cup granola (choose a low-sugar, moderate-carb option)
- 1 tablespoon honey (optional)

Instructions:

1. Arrange Greek yogurt, mixed berries, and granola in a glass or dish.
2. Drizzle with honey for extra sweetness if desired.
3. Enjoy your nutritious and satisfying parfait.

Total Calories:

- Approximately 300 calories

Preparation Time:

- 5 minutes

Sliced Apple with Almond Butter

Ingredients:

- 1 medium apple, sliced
- 2 tablespoons almond butter
- A sprinkle of cinnamon (optional)

Instructions:

1. Slice the apple into thin rounds or sticks.
2. Dip each apple slice into almond butter.
3. For extra flavor, sprinkle with a dash of cinnamon.

Total Calories:

- Approximately 250 calories

Preparation Time:

- 5 minutes

Caprese Skewers

Ingredients:

- Cherry tomatoes
- Fresh mozzarella balls
- Fresh basil leaves
- Balsamic vinegar and olive oil for drizzling
- Salt and pepper to taste

Instructions:

1. Skewer cherry tomatoes, fresh mozzarella balls, and fresh basil leaves onto toothpicks.
2. Drizzle over the olive oil and balsamic vinegar.
3. Add pepper and salt according to taste.

Total Calories:

- Approximately 200 calories

Preparation Time:

- 10 minutes

These moderate carb snack recipes offer a balance of carbohydrates, protein, and healthy fats to keep you satisfied and energized between meals on your moderate carb days. Enjoy these wholesome snack options while staying committed to your carb cycling plan.

Chapter 13

Moderate Carb Dessert Recipes

Satisfy your sweet tooth without straying from your moderate carb days with these delectable and balanced dessert recipes.

Baked Apples with Cinnamon

Ingredients:

- 2 apples (choose a moderate-carb variety like Granny Smith)
- 1 tablespoon unsalted butter
- 1 teaspoon ground cinnamon
- 2 tablespoons chopped walnuts
- 1 tablespoon honey (optional)

Instructions:

1. Preheat your oven to 375°F (190°C).
2. Core the apples, removing the seeds and a bit of the center to create a well.
3. Arrange the apples in a baking pan.
4. In a small bowl, mix the melted butter and ground cinnamon.
5. Drizzle the cinnamon butter over the apples.
6. If desired, fill the well of each apple with chopped walnuts and drizzle with honey.
7. Bake for 20-25 minutes or until the apples are tender.
8. Serve warm.

Total Calories:

- Approximately 250 calories per apple

Preparation Time:

- 30 minutes

Dark Chocolate-Dipped Strawberries

Ingredients:

- 6-8 fresh strawberries
- 2 oz dark chocolate (70% cocoa or higher)
- 1/2 teaspoon coconut oil
- Chopped nuts (e.g., almonds or walnuts) for garnish (optional)

Instructions:

1. Rinse and dry the strawberries thoroughly.
2. In a microwave-safe bowl, melt the dark chocolate and coconut oil in 20-second increments, stirring in between, until smooth.
3. Dip each strawberry into the melted chocolate, coating it halfway.
4. Place the dipped strawberries on a parchment paper-lined tray.
5. If desired, sprinkle chopped nuts over the chocolate-dipped portion.
6. Let the chocolate harden at room temperature or in the fridge before serving.

Total Calories:

- Approximately 80 calories per dipped strawberry

Preparation Time:

- 15 minutes

Chia Seed Pudding

Ingredients:

- 3 tablespoons chia seeds
- 1 cup unsweetened almond milk
- 1/2 teaspoon vanilla extract
- 1 tbsp low-carb sweetener (such as stevia or erythritol)
- Mixed berries for topping (e.g., blueberries, raspberries)

Instructions:

1. In a jar or bowl, combine chia seeds, almond milk, vanilla extract, and sweetener.
2. Stir well to disperse the chia seeds evenly.
3. Cover the jar or bowl and refrigerate for at least 3 hours or overnight, allowing the chia seeds to absorb the liquid and create a pudding-like consistency.
4. Before serving, top with mixed berries.

Total Calories:

- Approximately 200 calories

Preparation Time:

- 5 minutes (plus chilling time)

These moderate carb dessert recipes offer a balance of sweetness and nutrients, allowing you to indulge in a tasty treat while staying true to your carb cycling plan. Enjoy these delightful desserts during your moderate carb days.

Chapter 14

Moderate Carb Exercises

In this chapter, we'll explore the recommended exercises for your moderate carb days, providing detailed workout plans and valuable tips to make the most of your workouts while adhering to your carb cycling plan.

Recommended Exercises for Moderate Carb Days

- **Strength Training:** On moderate carb days, prioritize strength training exercises. This can include resistance training with free weights, resistance bands, or bodyweight exercises. Focus on compound movements like squats, deadlifts, bench presses, and lunges to work multiple muscle groups at once.

- **Cardiovascular Training:** Incorporate moderate-intensity cardio workouts like brisk walking, jogging, cycling, or swimming. This helps burn calories and improve cardiovascular health without depleting your glycogen stores.

- **Flexibility and Mobility Exercises:** Dedicate time to stretching and mobility exercises to improve flexibility and reduce the risk of injury. Pilates or yoga classes are great choices.

Detailed Workout Plans

Workout 1 - Full Body Strength Training:

- Squats: 3 sets of 8-10 reps
- Push-Ups: 3 sets of 10-12 reps
- Bent-Over Rows: 3 sets of 8-10 reps
- Planks: 3 sets of 30-45 seconds
- Rest: 45-60 seconds between sets

Workout 2 - Cardio and Core:

- 30 minutes of vigorous walking or running
- Cycling Crunches: 3 sets of 15-20 reps per side
- Leg Raises: Three sets of 10-12 reps
- Side Planks (each side): 3 sets of 30-45 seconds
- Rest: 30-45 seconds between core exercises

Workout 3 - Flexibility and Mobility:

- 20 minutes of yoga or Pilates
- Stretching exercises targeting major muscle groups
- Foam rolling to release muscle tension
- Deep breathing and relaxation techniques

Tips for Effective Moderate Carb Workouts

- **Stay Hydrated:** Proper hydration is crucial for energy and performance. Considerably drink water before, during, and after your exercise.
- **Pre-Workout Nutrition:** Consume a balanced meal or snack that includes carbohydrates, protein, and healthy fats 1-2 hours before your workout. This will provide the necessary fuel.
- **Progressive Overload:** Gradually increase the weight, intensity, or duration of your workouts to challenge your muscles and improve strength and endurance.
- **Protein Intake:** After your workout, have a protein-rich meal or snack to support muscle recovery and growth.
- **Mind-Body Connection:** Focus on proper form and technique during your exercises. Mindful movements can enhance your results and reduce the risk of injury.
- **Rest and Recovery:** Allow adequate time between exercises for your muscles to heal. Proper sleep is essential for overall health and performance.

By incorporating these exercises and following the workout plans, you'll maximize the benefits of your moderate carb days, maintain your energy levels, and support your overall fitness and health objectives. Staying consistent and making smart choices in your moderate carb workouts will help you reach your goals more effectively.

Part 3: High Carb Recipes and Exercises

In Part 3 of "Carb Cycling for Beginners," we'll explore high carb days, providing you with a variety of mouthwatering recipes and effective exercises designed for this phase of your carb cycling journey. High carb days are crucial for refilling your glycogen stores and providing the energy needed for intense workouts.

Chapter 15

High Carb Basics

In this chapter, we'll delve into the essential concepts of high carb days, providing you with a clear understanding of how this phase fits into your carb cycling journey.

Explanation of High Carb Days

High carb days are a pivotal element of your carb cycling plan. On these days, you will deliberately increase your carbohydrate intake to provide your body with a surge of energy, replenish glycogen stores, and fuel your workouts and physical activities.

The primary aim of high carb days is to enhance athletic performance, support muscle growth, and improve overall energy levels. These days are strategically placed in your carb cycling plan to ensure your body has the necessary resources to perform at its best.

Recommended Food Sources

To make the most of your high carb days, it's crucial to choose the right sources of carbohydrates. Focus on complex carbohydrates from wholesome, unprocessed foods. Some recommended food sources include:

- **Whole grains:** Brown rice, quinoa, whole wheat pasta, and oats.
- **Starchy vegetables:** Sweet potatoes, butternut squash, and peas.
- **Legumes:** Beans, lentils, and chickpeas.
- **Fruits:** Bananas, mangoes, and berries.
- **Dairy:** Greek yogurt and milk.
- **Lean proteins:** fish, tofu, turkey, and chicken.

These foods offer a rich source of nutrients, including carbohydrates, fiber, protein, and essential vitamins and minerals, ensuring you maintain optimal energy levels on your high carb days.

Benefits of High Carb Cycling

High carb cycling offers a range of benefits:

- **Enhanced Energy:** High carb days provide a substantial increase in available energy, ensuring you feel more energetic and can push harder during workouts.
- **Improved Exercise Performance:** With increased glycogen stores, your exercise performance and endurance improve, allowing you to lift more weight and perform longer cardio sessions.
- **Muscle Recovery and Growth:** The higher carbohydrate intake supports muscle recovery and growth, making high carb days ideal for resistance training.
- **Sustainable Energy:** High carb days provide sustained energy throughout the day, reducing fatigue and supporting overall well-being.

How to Calculate Your Daily Carb Intake on High Carb Days

Calculating your daily carbohydrate intake on high carb days is essential to tailor your carb cycling plan to your individual needs. Here's a simplified method:

- Determine your total daily calorie intake for weight maintenance or your specific goal (e.g., weight loss, muscle gain).
- On high carb days, aim to allocate about 50-60% of your total calories from carbohydrates. The exact percentage may vary based on your preferences and goals.
- Convert the calories from carbohydrates into grams. Carbohydrates provide approximately 4 calories per gram. For example, if you're consuming 2,000 calories per day, and you want 55% of those calories to come from carbohydrates, it would be (0.55 * 2,000) / 4 = 275 grams of carbohydrates.

By following these principles, you can personalize your carb intake on high carb days to align with your objectives and activity level while maintaining a balanced approach to nutrition and exercise.

Chapter 16

High Carb Breakfast Recipes

Kickstart your high carb day with a burst of energy by trying these delicious and nutritious high carb breakfast recipes.

Banana and Nut Butter Oatmeal

Ingredients:

- 1/2 cup rolled oats
- 1 cup almond milk (or any other kind of milk you like)
- 1 ripe banana, sliced
- 1 tablespoon nut butter (e.g., almond, peanut, or cashew)
- 1 tablespoon honey (optional)
- A sprinkle of cinnamon

Instructions:

1. Place almond milk and rolled oats in a saucepan. Stirring constantly, bring to a simmer.
2. Stir and cook for about 5 minutes or until the oats are creamy and cooked to your liking.
3. Pour the oatmeal into a bowl and top with sliced bananas, nut butter, a drizzle of honey, and a sprinkle of cinnamon.
4. Enjoy your hearty and energizing breakfast.

Total Calories:

- Approximately 400 calories

Preparation Time:

- 10 minutes

Fruit and Yogurt Parfait

Ingredients:

- 1/2 cup Greek yogurt
- 1/4 cup granola (choose a high-carb, low-sugar option)
- 1/2 cup of berries (strawberries, blueberries, raspberries e.t.c)
- 1/2 ripe mango, diced
- 1 tablespoon honey (optional)

Instructions:

1. In a glass or bowl, layer Greek yogurt, granola, mixed berries, and diced mango.
2. Drizzle with honey for extra sweetness if desired.
3. Enjoy your high-carb and satisfying parfait.

Total Calories:

- Approximately 350 calories

Preparation Time:

- 5 minutes

Sweet Potato Hash with Eggs

Ingredients:

- 1 medium peeled and sliced sweet potato
- 2 eggs
- 1/4 cup diced red bell pepper
- 1/4 cup diced onion
- 1/4 cup diced zucchini
- 1 tablespoon olive oil
- Salt and pepper to taste

Instructions:

1. In a pan over medium heat, warm the olive oil.
2. Add the diced sweet potato and sauté until it's slightly crispy and cooked through, about 8-10 minutes.
3. Add the red bell pepper, onion, and zucchini, and cook for an additional 5 minutes until the vegetables are tender.
4. Create two small wells in the mixture and crack an egg into each well.
5. Cover the skillet and cook until the egg whites are set but the yolks are still runny, about 3-5 minutes.
6. To taste, add salt and pepper for seasoning.
7. Serve your sweet potato hash with eggs.

Total Calories:

- Approximately 450 calories

Preparation Time:

- 20 minutes

These high carb breakfast recipes offer a balanced and nutritious start to your day, providing you with the energy you need for your high-intensity workouts and activities. Enjoy a variety of these breakfast options during your high carb days.

Chapter 17

High Carb Lunch Recipes

Lunch is the perfect time to refuel your energy for the rest of the day on your high carb day. Here are some mouthwatering high carb lunch recipes to keep you going.

Veggie and Quinoa Salad

Ingredients:

- 1 cup cooked quinoa
- 1/2 cup chickpeas, drained and rinsed
- 1/2 cup diced cucumbers
- 1/2 cup cherry tomatoes, halved
- 1/4 cup diced red onions
- 1/4 cup crumbled feta cheese
- Fresh parsley, chopped
- To dress, lemon juice and olive oil
- Salt and pepper to taste

Instructions:

1. In a bowl, combine cooked quinoa, chickpeas, cucumbers, cherry tomatoes, red onions, and feta cheese.
2. Drizzle with olive oil and lemon juice for dressing.
3. Toss the salad and season with salt and pepper.
4. Top with freshly chopped parsley.

Total Calories:

- Approximately 500 calories

Preparation Time:

- 15 minutes

Classic PB&J Sandwich with a Twist

Ingredients:

- 2 slices of whole-grain bread
- 2 tablespoons peanut butter
- 2 tablespoons fruit preserves or jelly (choose a high-carb variety)
- Sliced bananas or strawberries for extra filling

Instructions:

1. Spread peanut butter on one slice of bread and fruit preserves or jelly on the other.
2. Add sliced bananas or strawberries in the middle.
3. Put the two slices of bread together to make a satisfying PB&J sandwich.

Total Calories:

- Approximately 450 calories

Preparation Time:

- 5 minutes

Classic PB&J Sandwich with a Twist

Lentil and Vegetable Soup

Ingredients:

- 1 cup red lentils
- 1 carrot, diced
- 1 celery stalk, chopped
- 1 small onion, diced
- 1 garlic clove, minced
- 4 cups vegetable broth
- 1 teaspoon cumin
- 1/2 teaspoon paprika
- Salt and pepper to taste

Instructions:

1. In a large pot, sauté the diced onion, carrot, and celery until they soften.
2. Add minced garlic, cumin, and paprika, and cook for another minute.
3. Add red lentils and vegetable broth. Bring to a boil, then reduce the heat and simmer for 20-25 minutes or until the lentils are soft and the soup has thickened.
4. To taste, add salt and pepper for seasoning.
5. Serve your lentil and vegetable soup hot.

Total Calories:

- Approximately 400 calories

Preparation Time:

- 35 minutes

These high carb lunch recipes provide the energy you need to power through your day, whether you're at work, at the gym, or enjoying outdoor activities. Enjoy these wholesome and filling lunch options during your high carb days.

Chapter 18

High Carb Dinner Recipes

Dinner on your high carb days should be both satisfying and replenishing, ensuring you have the energy you need for your evening workouts and activities. Here are some delectable high carb dinner recipes for you to enjoy.

Chicken and Sweet Potato Curry

Ingredients:

- 8 oz chicken breast, cubed
- 1 sweet potato, peeled and diced
- 1/2 onion, chopped, 1 clove garlic, minced
- 1 tablespoon curry powder, 1 cup coconut milk
- Salt and pepper to taste
- Fresh cilantro for garnish
- Cooked brown rice (for serving)

Instructions:

1. In a large skillet, sauté the chopped onion and minced garlic until fragrant.
2. Add the chicken cubes and cook until they start to brown.
3. Stir in the diced sweet potato and curry powder.
4. Pour in the coconut milk and let the mixture simmer for 20-25 minutes, or until the sweet potatoes are tender.
5. Season with salt and pepper.
6. Serve your chicken and sweet potato curry over cooked brown rice and garnish with fresh cilantro.

Total Calories:

- Approximately 500 calories

Preparation Time:

- 40 minutes

Black Bean and Veggie Quesadillas

Ingredients:

- 4 whole-grain tortillas
- 1 can of rinsed black beans
- 1 cup finely chopped red, green, or yellow bell peppers
- 1 cup diced zucchini
- 1 cup shredded cheese (choose a moderate-carb variety)
- Olive oil for cooking
- Salsa and Greek yogurt for dipping

Instructions:

1. In a large skillet, sauté the diced bell peppers and zucchini until they're tender.
2. Remove the vegetables and set them aside.
3. In the same skillet, add a bit of olive oil and place one tortilla.
4. On the tortilla, layer black beans, sautéed vegetables, and shredded cheese.
5. Top with a second tortilla.
6. Cook for about 2-3 minutes on each side, or until the quesadilla is golden and the cheese is melted.
7. Continue with the remainder of the tortillas and fillings.
8. Cut each quesadilla into quarters and serve with salsa and Greek yogurt for dipping.

Total Calories:

- Approximately 450 calories

Preparation Time:

- 30 minutes

Spaghetti with Lentil Bolognese

Ingredients:

- 1 cup of brown lentils or dry green
- 8 oz whole-grain spaghetti
- 1 can crushed tomatoes
- 1 carrot, diced
- 1 celery stalk, chopped
- 1 onion, chopped
- 2 cloves garlic, minced
- 1 teaspoon dried oregano
- 1 teaspoon dried basil
- Salt and pepper to taste
- Fresh basil for garnish

Instructions:

1. Cook the lentils according to package instructions until they are tender.
2. Cook the whole-grain spaghetti according to package instructions and set aside.
3. In a large skillet, sauté the chopped onion, carrot, and celery until they soften.
4. Add minced garlic, dried oregano, and dried basil and cook for another minute.
5. Stir in the cooked lentils and crushed tomatoes.
6. Simmer for 15-20 minutes until the flavors meld together.
7. Season with salt and pepper.
8. Serve your lentil Bolognese sauce over the whole-grain spaghetti and garnish with fresh basil.

Total Calories:

- Approximately 550 calories

Preparation Time:

- 40 minutes

These high carb dinner recipes offer a combination of complex carbohydrates, proteins, and nutrients, ensuring you have the energy to tackle your evening workouts and enjoy your activities. Enjoy these wholesome and delicious dinner options during your high carb days.

Chapter 19

High Carb Snack Recipes

Maintain your energy levels between meals on your high carb days with these satisfying and delicious high carb snacks.

Rice Cakes with Nut Butter and Banana

Ingredients:

- 2 rice cakes
- 2 tablespoons nut butter (e.g., almond or peanut butter)
- 1 ripe banana, sliced
- A drizzle of honey (optional)

Instructions:

1. Spread nut butter evenly on the rice cakes.
2. Top with sliced bananas.
3. If desired, drizzle with honey for extra sweetness.

Total Calories:

- Approximately 350 calories

Preparation Time:

- 5 minutes

Trail Mix with Dried Fruits and Nuts

Ingredients:

- 1/4 cup mixed dried fruits (e.g., apricots, raisins, cranberries)
- 1/4 cup of mixed nuts (almonds, walnuts, cashews e.t.c)
- 2 tablespoons dark chocolate chips (70% cocoa or higher)

Instructions:

1. In a bowl, combine the dried fruits, mixed nuts, and dark chocolate chips.
2. Mix well.
3. Portion into snack-sized bags for convenient on-the-go snacking.

Total Calories:

- Approximately 400 calories per serving

Preparation Time:

- 5 minutes

Fruit Smoothie

Ingredients:

- 1 cup Greek yogurt
- 1/2 cup of berries (strawberries, blueberries, raspberries e.t.c)
- 1 ripe banana
- 1/2 cup orange juice
- 1 tablespoon honey (optional)

Instructions:

1. Blend Greek yogurt, mixed berries, ripe banana, and orange juice until smooth.
2. If desired, add honey for extra sweetness.
3. Pour into a glass and enjoy your refreshing high carb smoothie.

Total Calories:

- Approximately 350 calories

Preparation Time:

- 5 minutes

These high carb snack recipes are convenient, delicious, and provide the energy needed to power through your day. Enjoy these snacks while staying committed to your high carb days and carb cycling plan.

Chapter 20

High Carb Dessert Recipes

End your high carb day on a sweet note with these delectable high carb dessert recipes that will satisfy your cravings.

Banana and Blueberry Pancakes

Ingredients:

- 1 ripe banana, mashed
- 1/2 cup rolled oats
- 1/2 cup blueberries
- 1 egg
- 1/2 teaspoon vanilla extract
- A pinch of salt
- Maple syrup for drizzling (optional)

Instructions:

1. In a bowl, combine the mashed banana, rolled oats, blueberries, egg, vanilla extract, and a pinch of salt.
2. Mix until well combined.
3. In a nonstick skillet, heat the oil over medium heat.
4. Pour a ladleful of the batter onto the skillet to form a pancake.
5. Cook until bubbles form on the surface, then flip and cook until golden brown on both sides.
6. Serve with a drizzle of maple syrup if desired.

Total Calories:

- Approximately 400 calories

Preparation Time:

- 15 minutes

Mixed Berry Parfait with Granola

Ingredients:

- 1/2 cup Greek yogurt
- 1/2 cup of berries (strawberries, blueberries, raspberries e.t.c)
- 1/4 cup high-carb granola
- 1 tablespoon honey (optional)

Instructions:

1. Arrange Greek yogurt, granola, and mixed berries in a glass or dish.
2. Drizzle with honey for extra sweetness if desired.
3. Enjoy your high carb parfait.

Total Calories:

- Approximately 350 calories

Preparation Time:

- 5 minutes

Mixed Berry Parfait with Granola

Sweet Potato Brownies

Ingredients:

- 1 cup mashed sweet potatoes
- 1/2 cup almond butter
- 1/4 cup honey
- 1 egg
- 1/4 cup unsweetened cocoa powder
- 1/2 teaspoon baking soda
- 1/2 teaspoon vanilla extract
- A pinch of salt
- 1/4 cup chocolate chips (70% cocoa or higher)

Instructions:

1. Preheat your oven to 350°F (175°C) and grease a baking dish.
2. In a bowl, mix the mashed sweet potatoes, almond butter, honey, egg, cocoa powder, baking soda, vanilla extract, and a pinch of salt until smooth.
3. Fold in the chocolate chips.
4. Fill the baking dish with batter after greasing it.
5. Bake until a toothpick inserted into the middle comes out clean, 25 to 30 minutes.
6. Allow the brownies to cool before slicing and serving.

Total Calories:

- Approximately 400 calories

Preparation Time:

- 45 minutes

These high carb dessert recipes are a delightful way to conclude your high carb day. Savor these sweet treats while staying on track with your carb cycling plan.

Chapter 21

High Carb Exercises

High carb days are all about maximizing your energy for intense workouts. In this chapter, we'll explore the recommended exercises, provide detailed workout plans, and offer valuable tips for getting the most out of your high carb workouts.

Recommended Exercises for High Carb Days

- **High-Intensity Interval Training (HIIT):** HIIT workouts are ideal for high carb days because they can help you burn a significant amount of energy and improve your cardiovascular fitness in a short amount of time. These workouts typically involve short bursts of intense exercise followed by brief rest periods.

- **Resistance Training:** Incorporate resistance training to focus on muscle growth and strength. To work various muscular groups, you may employ bodyweight workouts, equipment, or free weights. High carb days provide the energy needed for challenging lifting sessions.

- **Sports and Athletic Activities:** Engage in team sports, solo sports, or athletic activities you enjoy, such as soccer, basketball, tennis, or swimming. These activities allow you to make the most of your increased energy levels.

Detailed Workout Plans

Workout 1 - High-Intensity Interval Training (HIIT):

- Jumping Jacks: 30 seconds
- Push-Ups: 30 seconds
- Mountain Climbers: 30 seconds
- Burpees: 30 seconds
- Rest: 60 seconds
- Repeat for 3 rounds

Workout 2 - Resistance Training: Full Body:

- Squats: 3 sets of 8-10 reps
- Deadlifts: 3 sets of 8-10 reps
- Bench Press: 3 sets of 8-10 reps
- Pull-Ups: 3 sets to failure
- Rest: 60-90 seconds between sets

Workout 3 - Sport-Specific Training: Tennis

- Tennis Practice: 30 minutes
- Footwork Drills: 10 minutes
- Rest: As needed during drills

Tips for Effective High Carb Workouts

- **Pre-Workout Meal:** Have a balanced meal containing carbohydrates, proteins, and healthy fats 1-2 hours before your workout. This provides fuel for your session.

- **Stay Hydrated:** Proper hydration is critical for high-intensity exercise. Considerably drink water before, during, and after your exercise.

- **Warm-Up:** Begin your workouts with a proper warm-up to prepare your muscles and prevent injury.

- **Post-Workout Nutrition:** After your workout, refuel with a meal rich in carbohydrates and protein to aid recovery and muscle growth.

- **Monitor Energy Levels:** Pay attention to how your body responds to the increased carb intake. Adjust your exercise intensity and duration accordingly.

- **Rest and Recovery:** Ensure you get enough rest and sleep to support muscle repair and overall well-being.

By following these exercises and workout plans, along with the provided tips, you'll make the most of your high carb days and achieve your fitness goals while maintaining a balanced approach to nutrition and exercise.

Meal-Exercise Plan

A comprehensive 30-day meal plan combining low, moderate, and high carb days

&

Detailed workout plans for the entire 30-day cycle

Chapter 22

A comprehensive 30-day meal plan

Below is a 30-day meal plan that combines low, moderate, and high carb days. This plan is designed to help you achieve your weight loss, muscle-building, and overall health goals through carb cycling. Please note that you can adjust portion sizes and ingredient choices based on your dietary preferences and specific calorie requirements.

Day 1: Low Carb

- Breakfast: Scrambled eggs with spinach and tomatoes.
- Lunch: Grilled chicken breast with a side of mixed greens.
- Snack: Greek yogurt with berries.
- Dinner: Baked salmon with asparagus.

Day 2: Moderate Carb

- Breakfast: Oatmeal with sliced banana and a spoon of almond butter.
- Lunch: Quinoa and black bean salad with veggies.
- Snack: Sliced apples with peanut butter.
- Dinner: Grilled shrimp with brown rice and broccoli.

Day 3: High Carb

- Breakfast: Greek yogurt parfait topped with mixed berries and granola.
- Lunch: Whole-grain bread with a turkey and avocado sandwich.
- Snack: Trail mix with nuts and dried fruits.
- Dinner: Spaghetti with whole-grain pasta and a side salad.

Day 4: Low Carb

- Breakfast: Cottage cheese with sliced peaches.
- Lunch: Tuna salad with mixed greens.
- Snack: Cucumber and bell pepper slices with hummus.
- Dinner: Grilled chicken with sautéed spinach.

Day 5: Moderate Carb

- Breakfast: Whole-grain waffles with Greek yogurt and strawberries.
- Lunch: Lentil and vegetable soup.
- Snack: Sliced pears with cheese.
- Dinner:Baked tilapia with quinoa and green beans.

Day 6: High Carb

- Breakfast: maple syrup and blueberries on pancakes.
- Lunch: Brown rice bowl with grilled tofu and stir-fried vegetables.
- Snack: Almond butter and banana slices on rice cakes.
- Dinner: Teriyaki chicken with jasmine rice.

Day 7: Low Carb

- Breakfast: Eggs scrambled with mushrooms and sautéed spinach.
- Lunch: Salad with grilled steak and balsamic vinaigrette.
- Snack: Hummus-topped celery and carrot sticks.
- Dinner: Roasted pork loin with steamed broccoli.

Day 8: Moderate Carb

- Breakfast: Oatmeal with sliced banana and a spoon of almond butter.
- Lunch: Quinoa and black bean salad with veggies.
- Snack: Sliced apples with peanut butter.
- Dinner: Grilled shrimp with brown rice and broccoli.

Day 9: High Carb

- Breakfast:** Greek yogurt parfait topped with mixed berries and granola.
- Lunch: Whole-grain bread with a turkey and avocado sandwich.
- Snack: Trail mix with nuts and dried fruits.
- Dinner: Spaghetti with whole-grain pasta and a side salad.

Day 10: Low Carb

- Breakfast: Cottage cheese with sliced peaches.
- Lunch: Tuna salad with mixed greens.
- Snack: Cucumber and bell pepper slices with hummus.
- Dinner: Grilled chicken with sautéed spinach.

Day 11: Moderate Carb

- Breakfast: Whole-grain waffles with Greek yogurt and strawberries.
- Lunch: Lentil and vegetable soup.
- Snack: Sliced pears with cheese.
- Dinner: Baked tilapia with quinoa and green beans.

Day 12: High Carb

- Breakfast: Maple syrup and blueberries on pancakes.
- Lunch: Brown rice bowl with grilled tofu and stir-fried vegetables.
- Snack: Almond butter and banana slices on rice cakes.
- Dinner: Teriyaki chicken with jasmine rice.

Day 13: Low Carb

- Breakfast: Scrambled eggs paired with mushrooms and sautéed spinach.
- Lunch: Salad with grilled steak and balsamic vinaigrette.
- Snack: Hummus-topped celery and carrot sticks.
- Dinner: Roasted pork loin with steamed broccoli.

Day 14: Moderate Carb

- Breakfast: Oatmeal with sliced banana and a spoon of almond butter.
- Lunch: Quinoa and black bean salad with veggies.
- Snack: Sliced apples with peanut butter.
- Dinner: Grilled shrimp with brown rice and broccoli.

Day 15: High Carb

- Breakfast: Greek yogurt parfait topped with mixed berries and granola.
- Lunch: Whole-grain bread toasted with turkey and avocado.
- Snack: Dried fruits and nuts mixed into trail mix.
- Dinner: Spaghetti with whole-grain pasta and a side salad.

Day 16: Low Carb

- Breakfast: Cottage cheese with sliced peaches.
- Lunch: Tuna salad with mixed greens.
- Snack: Cucumber and bell pepper slices with hummus.
- Dinner: Grilled chicken with sautéed spinach.

Day 17: Moderate Carb

- Breakfast: Whole-grain waffles with Greek yogurt and strawberries.
- Lunch: Lentil and vegetable soup.
- Snack: Sliced pears with cheese.
- Dinner: Baked tilapia with quinoa and green beans.

Day 18: High Carb

- Breakfast: Blueberry and maple syrup pancakes.
- Lunch: Stir-fried veggies and grilled tofu served in a brown rice bowl.
- Snack: Almond butter and banana slices on rice cakes.
- Dinner: Teriyaki chicken with jasmine rice.

Day 19: Low Carb

- Breakfast: Eggs scrambled with mushrooms and sautéed spinach.
- Lunch: Salad with grilled steak and balsamic vinaigrette.
- Snack: Hummus-topped carrot and celery sticks.
- Dinner: Roasted pork loin with steamed broccoli.

Day 20: Moderate Carb

- Breakfast: Oatmeal with sliced banana and a spoon of almond butter.
- Lunch: Quinoa and black bean salad with veggies.
- Snack: Sliced apples with peanut butter.
- Dinner: Grilled shrimp with brown rice and broccoli.

Day 21: High Carb

- Breakfast: Greek yogurt parfait topped with mixed berries and granola.
- Lunch: Whole-grain bread toasted with turkey and avocado.
- Snack: Dried fruits and nuts mixed into trail mix.
- Dinner: Spaghetti with whole-grain pasta and a side salad.

Day 22: Low Carb

- Breakfast: Cottage cheese with sliced peaches.
- Lunch: Tuna salad with mixed greens.
- Snack: Cucumber and bell pepper slices with hummus.
- Dinner: Grilled chicken with sautéed spinach.

Day 23: Moderate Carb

- Breakfast: Whole-grain waffles with Greek yogurt and strawberries.
- Lunch: Lentil and vegetable soup.
- Snack: Sliced pears with cheese.
- Dinner: Baked tilapia with quinoa and green beans.

Day 24: High Carb

- Breakfast: Maple syrup and blueberries on pancakes.
- Lunch: Brown rice bowl with grilled tofu and stir-fried vegetables.
- Snack: Almond butter and banana slices on rice cakes.
- Dinner: Teriyaki chicken with jasmine rice.

Day 25: Low Carb

- Breakfast: Eggs scrambled with mushrooms and sautéed spinach.
- Lunch: Salad with grilled steak and balsamic vinaigrette.
- Snack: Hummus-topped carrot and celery sticks.
- Dinner: Roasted pork loin with steamed broccoli.

Day 26: Moderate Carb

- Breakfast: Oatmeal with sliced banana and a spoon of almond butter.
- Lunch: Quinoa and black bean salad with veggies.
- Snack: Sliced apples with peanut butter.
- Dinner: Grilled shrimp with brown rice and broccoli.

Day 27: High Carb

- Breakfast: Greek yogurt parfait topped with mixed berries and granola.
- Lunch: Whole-grain bread toasted with turkey and avocado.
- Snack: Dried fruits and nuts mixed into trail mix.
- Dinner: Spaghetti with whole-grain pasta and a side salad.

Day 28: Low Carb

- Breakfast: Cottage cheese with sliced peaches.
- Lunch: Tuna salad with mixed greens.
- Snack: Cucumber and bell pepper slices with hummus.
- Dinner: Grilled chicken with sautéed spinach.

Day 29: Moderate Carb

- Breakfast: Whole-grain waffles with Greek yogurt and strawberries.
- Lunch: Lentil and vegetable soup.
- Snack: Sliced pears with cheese.
- Dinner: Baked tilapia with quinoa and green beans.

Day 30: High Carb

- Breakfast: Maple syrup and blueberries on pancakes.
- Lunch: Brown rice bowl with grilled tofu and stir-fried vegetables.
- Snack: Almond butter-topped rice cakes with banana slices.
- Dinner: Teriyaki chicken with jasmine rice.

This concludes your 30-day meal plan that combines low, moderate, and high carb days. You've successfully completed the program, and your balanced approach to nutrition will help you achieve your weight loss, muscle-building, and overall health goals through carb cycling. Continue to adjust portion sizes and ingredient choices as needed to meet your specific dietary preferences and calorie requirements. Congratulations on your commitment to your health and fitness journey!

Chapter 23

Workout plans for the entire 30-day cycle

Here's a 30-day exercise plan that combines a variety of workouts for low, moderate, and high carb days. Each workout is described with sets and repetitions to help you achieve your fitness goals.

Day 1: Low Carb - Strength Training

- Squats: 3 sets of 10 reps
- Push-Ups: 3 sets of 10 reps
- Lunges: 3 sets of 10 reps per leg
- Planks: 3 sets of 30 seconds

Day 2: Moderate Carb - Cardio

- Run or jog: 30 minutes
- Jumping Jacks: Three (3) sets of 20 reps
- Bicycle Crunches: 3 sets of 15 repetitions each side

Day 3: High Carb - Sport Activity

- Tennis: Play singles or doubles for 45 minutes
- Agility Drills: 3 sets of ladder drills
- Squash: Play a game for 30 minutes

Day 4: Low Carb - Bodyweight Workout

- Push-Ups: 3 sets of 12 reps
- Bodyweight Squats: 3 sets of 12 reps
- Planks: 3 sets of 45 seconds
- Leg Raises: Three (3) sets of 10 reps

Day 5: Moderate Carb - Interval Training

- Warm-up: 5 minutes of light jogging
- Sprint: 30 seconds
- Walk: 60 seconds (recovery)
- Repeat: 10 times
- Cool down: 5 minutes of walking

Day 6: High Carb - Active Rest

- Rest or engage in light activities like walking, stretching, or yoga.

Day 7: Low Carb - Strength Training

- Deadlifts: 3 sets of 8 reps
- Pull-Ups: 3 sets to failure
- Bent-Over Rows: Three (3) sets of 10 reps
- Russian Twists: 3 sets of 15 reps per side

Day 8: Moderate Carb - Cardio and Core

- Run or jog: 30 minutes
- Mountain Climbers: 3 sets of 15 reps per side
- Planks: 3 sets of 45 seconds

Day 9: High Carb - Sport Activity

- Play a team sport like soccer or basketball for 45 minutes.
- Agility Drills: 3 sets of cone drills or ladder drills.

Day 10: Low Carb - Strength Training

- Bench Press: Three (3) sets of 10 reps
- Dumbbell Lunges: 3 sets of 10 reps per leg
- Pull-Ups: 3 sets to failure
- Russian Twists: 3 sets of 20 reps (use a medicine ball if available)

Day 11: Moderate Carb - Interval Training

- Warm-up: 5 minutes of light jogging
- Sprint: 30 seconds
- Walk: 60 seconds (recovery)
- Repeat: 10 times
- Cool down: 5 minutes of walking

Day 12: High Carb - Sport Activity

- Engage in a high-intensity sport activity of your choice for 45 minutes.
- Agility Drills: 3 sets of agility ladder drills.

Day 13: Low Carb - Bodyweight Workout

- Push-Ups: 3 sets of 12 reps
- Bodyweight Squats: Three (3) sets of 15 reps
- Planks: 3 sets of 60 seconds
- Leg Raises: Three (3) sets of 12 reps

Day 14: Moderate Carb - Cardio and Core

- Swim: 30 minutes (if available)
- Bicycle Crunches: 3 sets of 20 repetitions each side
- Planks: 3 sets of 60 seconds

Day 15: High Carb - Sport Activity

- Play a game of your favorite high-intensity sport for 45 minutes.
- Agility Drills: 3 sets of cone drills or ladder drills.

Day 16: Low Carb - Strength Training

- Deadlifts: 3 sets of 8 reps
- Pull-Ups: 3 sets to failure
- Bent-Over Rows: 3 sets of 12 reps
- Russian Twists: 3 sets of 20 reps (use a medicine ball if available)

- **Day 17: Moderate Carb - Interval Training**
- Warm-up: 5 minutes of light jogging
- Sprint: 30 seconds
- Walk: 60 seconds (recovery)
- Repeat: 10 times
- Cool down: 5 minutes of walking

Day 18: High Carb - Active Rest

- Engage in light activities like walking, stretching, or yoga.

Day 19: Low Carb - Bodyweight Workout

- Push-Ups: 3 sets of 15 reps
- Bodyweight Squats: Three (3) sets of 15 reps
- Planks: 3 sets of 60 seconds
- Leg Raises: Three (3) sets of 15 reps

Day 20: Moderate Carb - Cardio and Core

- Run or jog: 30 minutes
- Bicycle Crunches: 3 sets of 20 repetitions each side
- Planks: 3 sets of 60 seconds

Day 21: High Carb - Sport Activity

- Participate in a high-intensity sport activity like tennis, basketball, or racquetball for 45 minutes.
- Agility Drills: 3 sets of cone drills or ladder drills.

Day 22: Low Carb - Strength Training

- Squats: 3 sets of 12 reps
- Push-Ups: 3 sets of 12 reps
- Lunges: 3 sets of 12 reps per leg
- Planks: 3 sets of 45 seconds

Day 23: Moderate Carb - Cardio

- Swim: 30 minutes (if available)
- Mountain Climbers: 3 sets of 20 reps per side
- Planks: 3 sets of 45 seconds

Day 24: High Carb - Sport Activity

- Engage in a sport or recreational activity of your choice for 45 minutes.
- Agility Drills: 3 sets of agility ladder drills.

Day 25: Low Carb - Bodyweight Workout

- Push-Ups: 3 sets of 15 reps
- Bodyweight Squats: Three (3) sets of 15 reps
- Planks: 3 sets of 60 seconds
- Leg Raises: Three (3) sets of 15 reps

Day 26: Moderate Carb - Interval Training

- Warm-up: 5 minutes of light jogging
- Sprint: 30 seconds
- Walk: 60 seconds (recovery)
- Repeat: 10 times
- Cool down: 5 minutes of walking

Day 27: High Carb - Active Rest

- Rest or engage in light activities like walking, stretching, or yoga.**

Day 28: Low Carb - Strength Training

- Deadlifts: 3 sets of 10 reps
- Pull-Ups: 3 sets to failure
- Bent-Over Rows: Three (3) sets of 15 reps
- Russian Twists: 3 sets of 20 reps (use a medicine ball if available)

Day 29: Moderate Carb - Cardio and Core

- Run or jog: 30 minutes

- Bicycle Crunches: 3 sets of 20 repetitions each side

- Planks: 3 sets of 60 seconds

Day 30: High Carb - Sport Activity

- Engage in a high-intensity sport or physical activity for 45 minutes.

- Agility Drills: 3 sets of cone drills or ladder drills.

This completes your 30-day exercise plan. The combination of strength training, cardio, and sport-specific activities is designed to help you achieve your fitness goals while aligning with your carb cycling plan. Be sure to prioritize proper form, rest, and hydration for the best results. Congratulations on your dedication to health and fitness!

Conclusion

Final Thought

In "Carb Cycling for Beginners," we've explored the intricacies of carb cycling, provided you with a wide array of recipes and effective exercise plans, and equipped you with valuable tips to help you achieve your weight loss, muscle-building, and overall health goals. Let's recap the key takeaways and encourage you to stay consistent on your journey.

Key Takeaways

- **Balanced Approach:** Carb cycling is a flexible approach that involves alternating between low, moderate, and high carb days to optimize energy, support muscle growth, and enhance weight management.
- **Nutrient-Dense Choices:** Emphasize whole, unprocessed foods, lean proteins, complex carbohydrates, and healthy fats to meet your dietary needs and maximize the benefits of carb cycling.
- **Energy Management:** Low carb days help promote fat loss, moderate carb days maintain a balance, and high carb days provide the energy for intense workouts and muscle growth.
- **Workout Variety:** Incorporate a variety of exercises, including strength training, cardio, and sport-specific activities, to target different fitness goals and keep your workouts engaging.
- **Meal Planning:** Meal planning and preparation are essential for success. By following the provided recipes and workout plans, you can stay on track with your carb cycling goals.

The Importance of Consistency

Consistency is the key to success in any fitness and nutrition journey. Regardless of the approach you choose, whether it's carb cycling or any other method, it's essential to stay dedicated to your goals. Here are a few reasons why consistency is vital:

- **Sustained Progress:** Consistency ensures that you make steady progress over time. Small, continuous efforts lead to significant results.
- **Habit Formation:** Consistency helps you form healthy habits. Over time, these habits become second nature and contribute to long-term success.

- **Adaptation:** Your body adapts to your routine, whether it's your workouts or your dietary choices. Consistency allows your body to adjust and optimize for your goals.
- **Motivation:** Seeing consistent progress can be a powerful motivator. It keeps you excited and committed to your journey.

Encouragement for Continued Progress

As you continue your carb cycling journey, remember that it's perfectly normal to face challenges along the way. Plateaus, cravings, and occasional setbacks are part of the process. The key is to stay positive, stay motivated, and make adjustments as needed. Here's some encouragement for your continued progress:

- **Stay Committed:** Your goals are worth the effort. Keep your vision clear and stay committed to your health and fitness journey.
- **Track Your Progress:** Keep a record of your workouts, meals, and how your body feels. This can help you make informed decisions and celebrate your achievements.
- **Seek Support:** Surround yourself with a support system, whether it's friends, family, or a fitness community. They can provide motivation and encouragement.
- **Flexibility:** Stay open to adjusting your plan when necessary. It's OK if a day doesn't go exactly as planned. How well you can adjust is what counts.
- **Appreciate Little Victories:** Celebrate and acknowledge the little accomplishments in your life. With each step you take, you grow closer to your goals.

With consistency, determination, and a balanced approach to nutrition and exercise, you can achieve the health and fitness outcomes you desire. Keep pushing forward on your carb cycling journey, and the results will speak for themselves.

www.ingramcontent.com/pod-product-compliance
Lightning Source LLC
Chambersburg PA
CBHW080823280726

48660CB00019B/3653